# DEDICATION

I would like to dedicate this book to all my prayer students and our Church The Residence of Christ Ministries Head Quarters in Mkushi – Zambia. I don't want to forget my Intercessors who stand in prayer for the ministry with a passion to see God's kingdom advancing.

# TABLE OF CONTENTS

Introduction



**About the Author**

# 10 KEYS TO HEALING

# AND GOOD HEALTH

**APOSTLE ARTHUR MUSONDA**

# PREFACE

The main purpose of this book is to help many Christians see how easy it is to receive healing for the sick and maintain good health. I will make it very easy to understand by bringing out scriptures that will instantly challenge you to get hold of the healing power of God for yourself or for others.

I have provided exercises/prayer at the end of each chapter to activate you in the healing anointing so that even as you're reading the book, you are praying and seeing the results. God's word is the standard I have followed to share everything I have discussed in this short book for that's where the power of God is (**Romans 1:16**). God's word is the truth. I will show you that you can live sickness and disease free no matter your now condition. Spiritual things are real and can be practiced by following simple and yet powerful steps found in God's word.

God has said in His word that whoever asks receives, whoever seeks finds and whoever knocks,

the door is opened for him/her (**Mathew 7:8**).
Therefore you just need to learn a few principles to
apply and you shall see the healing power of God
manifest. I will also share with you a few things I
have experienced myself concerning this subject. I
am a living testimony to what I am sharing with you
in this book. These keys have worked for me,
through me and through others. I believe by the
time you finish reading this book and doing the
exercises/prayers I have included, you will be
healed if you're sick, your faith will be lifted to
another level, and will you feel bold and anointed to
heal the sick. God bless you as you enjoy reading
this short book.

# Introduction

I would like to thank God that you are reading this book about your healing and good health. I didn't want to write a big book about healing because my intention is not to give a complicated theological in depths concerning this subject.  I want even a sick person, someone in pain or on the sick bed to understand in a simple and yet powerful way what is needed for them to receive their healing and maintain their good health. You don't have to spend many days to finish this book. I will ask you to apply every exercise I have put in the book so that even as you read, change will be evident in your life. Today thousands and millions of people die every year from many diseases and sickness and I know our dedicated scientists and medical doctors work tirelessly investigating and conducting many research studies around the world in order to find cures and disease prevention methods.

There are many scriptures that shows us God's promises that include our healing. You will find God saying things like "I will not bring upon you any of the diseases I brought upon the Egyptians, none shall be barren among you (Exodus 15:26, Deuteronomy 7:15) etc. Now I am not just dealing with God's promises in this lesson. There are just simple keys I am providing which will work for you easily to change your life. I know we could get into understanding this subject by digging into the Hebrew and Greek languages in exploring what certain scriptures say theologically but I don't intend to make it difficult, complicated or take most of your time as you learn about this subject. It's just all about simple things with exercises/prayers at the end of each chapter and that's it.

# Chapter One

# Knowledge - Key #1

*....there are things God cannot do not because He isn't powerful enough but because it's against the spiritual laws He instituted to govern certain operations especially when it comes to the invasion of the spiritual into the physical realm.*

Let us start by looking at **Hosea 4:6** where the bible says "***My people are destroyed for lack of knowledge: because thou hast rejected knowledge, I will also reject thee, that thou shalt be no priest to me: seeing thou hast forgotten the law of thy God, I will also forget thy children***" When I looked at this scripture, I realized that there are things God cannot do not because He isn't powerful enough but because it's against some spiritual laws He instituted to govern certain operations especially when it comes to the invasion of the spiritual into the physical realm. God has knowledge on everything and by His grace He has also provided us with what we must know to see us go to heaven and all we need for our earthily living. Manufactures of electrical appliances make sure they include the manual so that buyers can have knowledge on how to use the appliance to avoid accidents and also to just make sure the appliance is used correctly for it serve its purpose. This is very important also when it comes to spirituality. We need to know what God has said about our lives especially when we are here on earth. I know that we shall keep on learning even after we have gone to heaven but there is what we must know while we are here on earth. So now to be specific here, we are dealing with the subject of healing and good health. What has the bible said about our health? I have heard people pray wrong prayers because of lack of knowledge.  I remember one time about some 13 to 14 years ago we were praying during our Sunday service intercession prayers when I head in my spirit the Lord say to me "stop begging me to cast out the devil, use the authority you have and command the devil". I immediately told everyone to stop praying and told them to pray correctly. Many were asking God to cast out the devils that were against our service that day and the Lord helped us by telling us to pray the right way. I will discuss more about this in the chapter about authority.  At this point I want you to begin to think about how you pray about sickness or how you respond when you feel bad in your body or even when you hear that someone is sick. It all depends on the knowledge you have in your spirit and soul.

Let's also take a look at **2 Peter 1:3** which says that "***God has given us (past tense) all things that pertain to life and godliness through the knowledge of Him***". Notice the bible says "**through the knowledge of Him**". We gain access to what God has provided for us through knowledge. That is why I believe that through the knowledge you are gaining from this short lesson, you are having access as well to God's power that restores and gives life to the human body. Many people wait for God to do what they must do because they don't know they have a role to play. At this point now you need to know that the supernatural must be invited by us. According to the law of spirituality, man has authority to operate here on earth and can demand change by inviting the spiritual and therefore sitting and waiting for when things will change is just lack of knowledge. Waiting on God actually means positioning yourself spiritually and inviting God according to knowledge of the scriptures. So now we need to know what God has said about our health and body restoration or healing for us to claim our health. I have heard of people who when they are sick say things like "let's allow the will of God and if God wants to heal He will etc". When we read the bible, there are of course a number of people that God didn't want healed in the old covenant because the sickness was part of judgment.  Otherwise we must all know that is it God's will for us to be in good health so that we can accomplish that which He has purposed for our lives each one of us.

It is through the little knowledge I have received from God's word that God has been able to keep me from sicknesses and diseases. I believe it shall be so in your life also. So the key I am giving out in this chapter is that of knowledge. If you are a child of God, get this knowledge so that you don't perish. Sickness is not yours, it came because of sin which Jesus Christ has dwelt with on the cross. I believe this book will provide you with the knowledge you need to know for your health even as you continue to read.

## Exercise/Prayer

- ➤ My Father my maker in heaven, I worship you. Your name be blessed and praised forever.
- ➤ I declare today that the Holy Spirit open my spirit to understand things of the spirit in Jesus' name

- ➢ I pray that I shall not be ignorant about the privileges I have in Christ Jesus and the promises of God for my healing and health in the name of Jesus Christ.
- ➢ As I read your word and pray, let spiritual knowledge be imparted in my spirit for me to manifest what you say I am in Jesus' name I pray Amen.

# Chapter Two

## Origin of Sickness Dealt with - Key #2

Allow me to talk about where sickness came from in the first place so that you know where it belongs. And please let me also note that **I am not** sharing with you scientific findings and understanding about the origin of sickness. What we are dealing with here is spiritual. I want you to know and understand that sickness is not yours. It does not belong to your body and neither do you belong to it if you're a child of God. It came from somewhere and should be sent where it belongs.  I am a man of faith and I believe God so much that I don't limit him, I don't put God in a box. I believe He can do anything, any miracle, He can kill someone and bring them back to life again. God is God.

Now when I say origin is sickness, I also don't mean causes of sicknesses as described by medical doctors.  For instance, we know the mosquitos transmit malaria parasites that multiply in the body and cause many deaths around the world, however, what I am talking about here is more than that which doesn't even require medical equipment to change but your spirit, soul and body through faith and spiritual knowledge.

Let me begin by saying that there is a spiritual world from where this physical world came from. **Colossians 1:16** tells us how through Christ Jesus all things were created, both the visible and the invisible. And when Jesus rose from the dead, He ascended into the invisible world while His disciples watched. So if the visible came from the invisible, we must know that, the invisible is superior and that the physical world is controlled from the spiritual world. Now did God created sickness? The answer is no. Let's take a look at **Genesis 1:31** where the bible says "***God saw all that he had made, and it was very good. And there was evening, and there was morning—the sixth day***". Nothing was going to affect Adam and cause him sick or diseased. God created everything good.

Sickness is not good and it obviously didn't originate from God just like any other evil didn't. So then how did man begin to get sick and die? When we read the bible, we discover that it was the birth of sin that came with sickness, death and many other tribulations of this world and this wasn't the original plan of God. Satan brought in sin which gave birth to decay when man lost his place in the presence and fellowship of/with God. Sickness is a result of the sin of Adam and Eve. When it came in, man died spiritually, began to die physically and also began to get sick Romans 5:12 puts it this way ***"Therefore, just as sin entered the world through one man, and death through sin, and in this way death came to all people, because all sinned"***. Now when we become born again, we by faith receive forgiveness of sin and are spiritually restored in our fellowship with God. The issue of the sin of Adam was dealt with by our Lord Jesus Christ on the cross. Now if He dealt with this issue of sin (which He did of course) which introduced sickness, we must also by faith receive back our good health and every good thing Adam and Eve enjoyed before the fall. When you get born again by receiving Jesus as Lord of your life, you also receive restoration to God's original state of being of humans.

The conclusion here is that the devil brought sin through which man began to die and get sick. But our Lord Jesus (the second Adam-**1 Corinthians 15:45**) also came and took away sin through which we receive life and should be able to claim our healing and good health. I would also like to assume that you're born again and just want to learn more about living in good health and also helping others receive their healing. However in case you're not born again, allow me to lead you in a prayer of salvation below so that you have the benefits found in Christ Jesus and also gain access to God's healing power

**Pray this prayer**; *God in heaven my maker, I acknowledge being a sinner. I ask for your forgiveness and I believe that Jesus Christ died for*

*my sins and that God raised Him from the dead. Jesus Christ today I ask you to come in my heart and be my Lord and personal savior. Your blood carried away my sins and today I receive the washing away of my sins in Jesus' name. Today I declare I am a child of God Amen.* **(John 1:12).**

As God's children we are to avoid sin which we have learnt above as being the source of decay and sickness. In **John 5:5-14** the bibles tells this story "***One man there had been an invalid for thirty-eight years. When Jesus saw him lying there and realized that he had spent a long time in this condition, He asked him, "Do you want to get well?" "Sir," the invalid replied, "I have no one to help me into the pool when the water is stirred. While I am on my way, someone else goes in before me."Then Jesus told him, "Get up, pick up your mat, and walk."Immediately the man was made well, and he picked up his mat and began to walk.***

*Now this happened on the Sabbath day, so the Jews said to the man who had been healed, "This is the Sabbath! It is unlawful for you to carry your mat."But he answered, "The man who made me well told me, 'Pick up your mat and walk.'""Who is this man who told you to pick it up and walk?" they asked. But the man who was healed did not know who it was, for Jesus had slipped away while the crowd was there. Afterward, Jesus found the man at the temple and said to him, "See, you have been made well. Stop sinning, or something worse may happen to you"* We have to learn something from this. When the Lord Jesus said "**Stop sinning, or something worse may happen to you**" it means sin caused this man's condition such that if He continued living in sin, a worse condition was going to come his way. Now we must also understand that sin can cause sickness as well us hinder prayer from being answered and can also remove a person from a place of exercising authority. The devil can advantage of one's sin as a legal right to bring affliction for sin opens the door to demonic influences. You cannot be living in sin and yet you expect God almighty the holy one of heaven the creator of all to delight in healing you. When you have sinned you must be sorry to God, confess your sins and repent (not going back to sinning). The problem of sin has been dealt with by Jesus Christ on the cross therefore as a child of God, lay off every weight and every sin that easily entangles you. (**Hebrews 12:1**).

## Exercise/Prayer

> ➢ My Father my maker in heaven, I worship you. Your name be blessed and praised forever.
> ➢ I believe that you're a good God and everything you created was good. It was satan who brought in sin which brought in sickness.
> ➢ Father in heaven I am also sorry for every sin I have not repented of (mention the sin

before God in confession if there be any) and today I repent, I will not go back to sin again by your grace in Jesus' name

- ➢ Now because Jesus Christ took away sin which brought in sickness and because I am a child of God whose sins were paid for on the cross of Calvary by my Lord Jesus Christ, I claim and receive my healing and good health in Jesus' name. As I received salvation by believing with my heart and confessing Jesus Christ as my Lord and Savior, I receive restoration of my body in Jesus' name to function according your original plan
- ➢ I declare that no sickness and disease has a place in my body in Jesus' name Amen.

# Chapter Three

# God's will - Key #3

I want us to discuss the will of God concerning our health from the written word/will of God. I know also that there is still something God has to say prophetically about any man's current condition.  In everything God has something to say. When someone is sick, God always has a word about that situation and we must pray to get His opinion. However, that's not what we are talking about here. God's written word is to be our number one standard because even a prophetic word is always subject to the written word of God. It has to be consistent with the written word of God. We are also told from scripture to judge every prophecy (**1 Corinthians 14:29**) and we can do that using God's word which discerns the intents of the heart (**Heb 4:12**)

So now according the word of God, what do we find as God's will concerning healing and our health generally? I will start by saying "**it is God's will for every person to be healed and be in good health**". When we read the bible, we will see that God had provided a way out of sickness both in the old and new covenants, clearly showing us that God doesn't want us sick just as we have seen from the origin of sickness that God didn't bring it on mankind. God anoints men and woman with great healing power to heal the sick which means He wants us well. In this chapter, I will give you scriptures that show the will of God to heal and keep us in good health. Sicknesses and diseases have claimed the lives of so many people around the world. Some families have lost bread winners through sickness. There are people who had all the money they needed in life and yet sickness took their lives even after having received proper medical services the world can offer. Knowing the will of God concerning the problem of sickness is also key because miracles start from there.  We must know God's will concerning everything so that when we pray, we do it according to God's will. Look at this scripture "**_And this is the confidence that we have in him, that, if we ask any thing according to his will, he heareth us:_**

**_15 And if we know that he hear us, whatsoever we ask, we know that we have the petitions that we desired of him_**

**_"_** (**1 John 5:14-15**). So if your prayer is not according to God's will, it's empty and won't yield the desired results. Actually even faith is based on information which is God's will/word in this case and so when we pray according to that will of God, healing is guaranteed.

## God's will before Jesus Christ Came

Let me start by giving a few scriptures from God's word that shows us God's will concerning sickness before Jesus Christ came on earth.

- We start with Exodus 23:25. The bible says "**_And ye shall serve the LORD your God,_**

**and he shall bless thy bread, and thy water; and I will take sickness away from the midst of thee**". This meant serving God as we do as Christians today. God had promised to take away sickness from among His children and that is His will. He is willing to heal the sick and keep His children in good health.

- Isiah 53:4 – 5 "**Surely he took up our pain and bore our suffering, yet we considered him punished by God, stricken by him, and afflicted.[5] But he was pierced for our transgressions, he was crushed for our iniquities; the punishment that brought us peace was on him, and by his wounds we are healed**". I have used this scripture here even though the fulfilment of it came when Jesus Christ died and rose from the dead. This scripture shows how God planned it from the start to have our Lord Jesus Christ wounded for our healing. All of us living now were not even there when this took place. He suffered and was wounded for our healing even before we were born.

- Jeremiah 33:6 "***Nevertheless, I will bring health and healing to it; I will heal my people and will let them enjoy abundant peace and security***". God promised to bring healing and good health here. He doesn't want any of His children be afflicted with any sickness. He wants us all well. We can't enjoy life and accomplish what we were born for when we are afflicted with sicknesses and therefore God has always been willing to heal.

- Psalms 103:2 – 4 "***Praise the LORD, my soul, and forget not all his benefits, He who forgives all your iniquities and heals all your diseases, who redeems your life from the Pit and crowns you with loving devotion and compassion***". The scripture is talking about praising God and not forgetting His benefits. There are so many benefits in God and when you are His child, healing and good health is your benefit. The bible clearly shows us here that healing from diseases is one of the benefits found in being a child of God. Praise God! I love this scripture for I am a beneficiary of God's benefits.

- Psalms 41:2 – 3 "***The LORD will protect and preserve him; He will bless him in the land and refuse to surrender him to the will of his foes, The LORD will sustain him on his bed of illness and restore him from his bed of sickness***." Here we see God's will for His children when they are ill. He declared His desire and will to restore His children from sickbeds. There is a saying I have and it goes like this "**If God doesn't want it, I don't want it either**". Your will and prayer must align with God's will. If you know anyone who has been sick, preach these scripture to them and pray over them according to the will of God which is "**healing them and raising them from their sick beds**". Knowing all this about your health must give you boldness when you pray in Jesus' name.

## God's will during the ministry of Jesus Christ on earth

When Jesus Christ came on earth as "**Emmanuel**" meaning God with us (**Mathew 1:23**), what was the will of God concerning man's health? Did it change from what we have seen above before He came? Let us look at some scriptures;

- Luke 4:18 "***The Spirit of the Lord is upon me, for he has anointed me to bring Good News to the poor. He has sent me to proclaim that captives will be released, that the blind will see, that the oppressed will be set free***" When Jesus was baptized by John the Baptist, the Holy Spirit led Him into the wilderness to pray and fast for forty days, forty nights and it was after He finished that He declared what we read in the scripture above. While praying and fasting in the wilderness, I believe so many things took place such as supernatural encounters with the Father, angels and demons. The bible doesn't tell us much about that except the encounters He had with the devil who came to tempt him and angels coming to minister to Him. I believe it was during this time that a might anointing came upon him which He revealed in the above scripture. Now what is my main point here? God anointed Jesus to heal, open eyes of the blind etc, showing us His will to heal the sick. So God still demonstrated His will for man to live in good health.

- Mathew 4:23 – 24 "***Jesus went throughout Galilee, teaching in their synagogues, preaching the gospel of the kingdom, and healing every disease and sickness among the people, News about Him spread all over Syria, and people brought to Him all who were ill*** *with various diseases, those suffering acute pain, the demon-possessed, those having seizures, and the paralyzed—and He healed them"* Most of these scriptures are just self-explanatory. He went about healing every disease and sickness among the people. And I like it when the scripture says "**every disease and sickness**". There is no such a thing as curable or incurable disease when it comes to God's power. Whether it is HIV, cancer, diabetes, paralysis, God can heal every one of them and it is His will.

- Luke 13:11 – 13 "*and a woman there had been disabled by a spirit for eighteen years. She was hunched over and could not stand up straight, When Jesus saw her, He called her over and said, "Woman, you are set free from your infirmity, Then He laid His hands on her, and immediately she straightened up and began to glorify God'* Scriptures like this make my spirit soul and body move. The woman didn't even ask Jesus to heal her but He simply called her when He so her and said be healed. He laid His hands on her and she was healed instantly, my God! He doesn't want people sick and afflicted. He made us, created our bodies to function well in this world and when He saw this woman who couldn't move straight up, he released His power and healed her.

- Mathew10:1 "***Jesus called his twelve disciples to him and gave them authority to drive out impure spirits and to heal every disease and sickness***" Here we see our Lord Jesus giving power to the disciples against unclean spirits to cast them out and heal all manner of sickness and all manner of diseases. Now notice the bibles uses the word "**against**" and this means God is against demons, sickness and disease. So if anyone was wondering whether it is God's will to heal or not, get it from here also that

God is against sickness. He gives His
servants power which works against sickness
and disease to flash them out of human
bodies.

- Luke 5:12 - 13 "***In one of the villages,
Jesus met a man with an advanced case
of leprosy. When the man saw Jesus, he
bowed with his face to the ground,
begging to be healed. "Lord," he said,
"if you are willing, you can heal me and
make me clean, Jesus reached out His
hand and touched the man. "I am
willing," He said. "Be clean!" And
immediately the leprosy left him***" From
this scripture I can conclude that this man
wasn't sure of God's will concerning his
condition and therefore asked Jesus to heal
Him if at all He was willing and thank God
Jesus is always willing to heal. We cannot
pray like this man anymore because we now
know it is His will heal and keep us in good
health.  He is a good God always willing to

make us well and once our will becomes consistent with God's will, our body cells respond by being healed.

- Luke 5:17 "***One day Jesus was teaching, and Pharisees and teachers of the law were sitting there. They had come from every village of Galilee and from Judea and Jerusalem. And the power of the Lord was with Jesus to heal the sick***" In this meeting the Lord Jesus had, we see His power being present to heal the sick. He made His power to heal present in His meetings with the people. And even now when He is present in our midst, His healing power is ever present. He knew some sick people might be present in the meeting and therefore made His healing power available for it is His will to heal the sick. It might seem like I am repeating certain words and terms but I must let you know that repetition is the mother of learning and improvement. During meditation, we must think and talk about the same thing over and over until it gets even into our sub conscious.

- Mathew 14:14 "***When Jesus landed and saw a large crowd, he had compassion on them and healed their sick***" Healing is of the things Jesus did so much among the people and there are so many scriptures in all the four gospels that shows us that. He was moved with compassion and healed their sick. Even in our time, He gets moved in our meetings and heals the sick.

- Luke 4:38-40 "***Jesus left the synagogue and went to Simon's house. Simon's mother-in-law was very sick. She had a high fever. They asked Jesus to do something to help her. [39] He stood very close to her and ordered the sickness to go away. The sickness left her, and she got up and began serving them, [40] when the sun went down, the people brought their sick friends to Jesus. They had many different kinds of sicknesses.***

*Jesus laid his hands on each sick person and healed them all*' We see Peter's mother in-law afflicted with a high fever and when the people saw Jesus come to the house, they asked Him to do something about it and because it is His will to heal, He ordered the fever it leave and it left her immediately. Afterwards that same day we see many people begin to bring their sick to this house and Jesus didn't just heal one or heal some of the sick but all of them the bible says. He never wanted anyone of them be afflicted with sickness anymore. Even now God can heal every one that is sick and this is why I am giving out these simple and yet effective keys to activate God's healing power.

- Acts 10:38 "*how God anointed Jesus of Nazareth with the Holy Spirit and power, and how he went around doing good and healing all who were under the power of the devil, because God was with him*" Like we have discussed above in **Luke 4:18** about Jesus being anointed, here is another one. God the Father anointed Jesus Christ to do good which included healing people. God is good and does what is good and perfect. Our Lord Jesus carried anointing to perform many signs and wonders and healing was one of them because He is a God that cares and compassionate and wants us fit and well in our physical bodies.

## God's will after Jesus' Ascension

I want us now to see what the will of God is now that Jesus has already gone back to the Father. I will give a few scripture as well from the New Testament

- Mark 16:17 – 18 "**16 *And these signs will accompany those who believe: In my name they will drive out demons; they will speak in new tongues 16 they will pick up snakes with their hands, and if*** *__they drink any deadly poison, it will not harm them; they will lay their hands on the sick, and they will be made well__*'.

This wonderful scripture shows us that God is willing to make the sick well even now.  He said the manifestation of His healing power through the laying on of hands on the sick is one of the signs that will follow believers in Christ Jesus.  Even after Jesus died and rose from the dead, He declared through this scripture that healing of the sick is God's will and He provided a way out of sickness and not a way into it. And another thing I get from this scripture is that if believers shall be followed by a sign of laying hands on the sick making them healed, I see a suggestion that as believers in Christ Jesus we carry God's healing power in us which is transferred to the sick through the laying on of hands and we can also exercise the same power on ourselves to make live in good health. The believer is used by God to heal the sick and himself can stay without being sick. This may be hard for many to believe that a believer in Christ can stay without sickness.  Let me elaborate this further; Jesus said "**if they (believers in Christ) drink any deadly poison it shall not hurt them**" now what is poison? It's those things that eat up and kill the cells in the body! Things like bacteria, parasites, viruses, germs, chemicals etc. Of course we cannot take poison deliberately to prove the scripture for that will be foolishness and not faith! It's putting God to test when the bible says we shouldn't (**Luke 4:12**). We also see this demonstrated when the apostle Paul was accidentally bitten by a poisonous viper. Acts 28:3-6 "*3 Paul gathered a pile of brushwood and, as he put it on the fire, a viper, driven out by the heat, fastened itself on his hand. 4 When the islanders saw the snake hanging from his hand, they said to each other, "This man must be a* *murderer; for though he escaped from the sea, the goddess Justice has not allowed him to live.'* [5] *But Paul shook the snake off into the fire and suffered no ill effects.* [6] *The people expected him to swell up or suddenly fall dead; but after waiting a long time and seeing nothing unusual happen to him, they changed their minds and said he was a god'*. This is powerful and we should all desire and pray to walk in this kind of truth Jesus Christ released. Apostle Paul walked in it and it's available to us today. The people knew the snake was venomous and expected to see Paul drop dead, however he wasn't even worried and just continued doing what he was doing. The venom couldn't harm him. Isn't this supernatural? It is and it's for you and me. No matter what kind of infection come near, we are promised not to be hurt. Believe this for yourself right now in Jesus' name.

- Acts 9:33 – 34 "*There he found a man named Aeneas, who had been paralyzed and bedridden for eight years. "Aeneas," Peter said to him, "Jesus Christ heals you! Get up and put away your mat." Immediately Aeneas got up*,." Peter here was used by the Lord Jesus to heal Aeneas. Now Jesus already ascended to heaven and all what Peter said to the sick man was "**Jesus Christ heals you, Get up and roll your mat**" and the man was immediately restored. This means He is still healing even today. It is His will for you and me to live in good health.  You can say to yourself what Peter said to the sick like for instance "Jesus Christ makes me well, keeps my body well" etc.

- Acts 3:6 "*But Peter said, "Silver or gold I do not have, but what I have I give you: In the name of Jesus Christ of Nazareth, get up and walk*!" Peter again released healing power to this man's life when Jesus was in heaven just like He is today. See yourself as the Peter of today in this case and release the healing power of God to the sick. So my main point here is that even after Jesus has ascended to heaven, His will to heal the sick continues until He comes back.

- Romans 8:11 "**And if the Spirit of him who raised Jesus from the dead is living in you, he who raised Christ from the dead will also give life to your mortal bodies because of his Spirit who lives in you**". The bible now gives another way we can stay healed and stay in good health. And that is through the Holy Spirit dwelling in us. The Father through the power of the Holy Spirit raised Jesus from the dead and anyone with the Holy Spirit in them can access this resurrection power of God in their body

- 1 Corinthians 12:9 – 10 "**to another faith by the same Spirit, to another gifts of** *healing by that one Spirit, to another the working of miracles, to another prophecy, to another distinguishing between spirits, to another speaking in various tongues, and to still another the interpretation of tongues*" Here I just want to talk about God's will to heal the sick through the gifts of the Spirit He gives to men to heal. The Holy Spirit specially gifts believers with diversities of manifestations and some of which are healings and working of miracles. Meaning God still wants you well in your body even today. If healing wasn't' for today, God was not going to give healing gifts to men!

- 1 Peter 2:24 "*He himself bore our sins" in his body on the cross, so that we might die to sins and live for righteousness; "by his wounds you have been healed*" I love how this scripture puts it "**you have been healed**" in past tense. I have used this scripture confessing it over and over and have seen the fruit. It works because it was done and finished on the cross of Calvary. Jesus took away sin and sickness and you know what?, just as you can refuse to live in sin by hating it because God doesn't want it, you can also refuse to be sick because Jesus took away sickness as well through His wounds. This is reality, Jesus wasn't wounded for nothing it was for our healing and good health and even the devil knows that.

- James 5:14 "***Is anyone among you sick? Let them call the elders of the church to pray over them and anoint them with oil in the name of the Lord***' I will still discuss more about this scripture in another chapter when I talk about how love and forgiveness are connected with healing. However what I want to bring out here for now is the invitation to pray for the sick. God is saying healing awaits them that will pray, it is available in the name of Jesus Christ our

Lord and savior. The elders of the church mentioned here is not necessarily leaders of the church but the mature Christians who understand spiritual things and can offer prayers of faith. Therefore you can pray for yourself or the sick, have this in mind that God has invited us to pray and He will do the healing.

- 3 John 1:2 "***Beloved, I pray that in every way you may prosper and enjoy good health, as your soul also prospers***." I love this scripture because it plains say "**enjoy good health**" and that's what we all want in this world. No one wants to suffer with sickness and disease and neither does God want us sick. Prayer is mentioned in this scripture and I believe we can pray today asking God that we want to enjoy good health and all should go well with us. If it's a prayer point in the bible, then God already has the answer for it for the bible says "**the**

**promises of God are yes and amen in Christ** (Corinthians 1:20)".

## Same yesterday, today and forever

If God didn't create sickness, it was His will to heal the sick before Christ came, was His will to heal while He came as Emmanuel (**Mathew 1:23, John 1:14**) and after Jesus Christ ascended to heaven He continued to heal, we must be excited even today because Hebrews 13:8 says "**Jesus Christ is the same yesterday and today and forever**". If Jesus was moved with compassion and healed the sick, had His power present to heal the sick, told the leper "I am willing to make you well" He will do again today because he never changes. He is the same compassionate God full of love and always willing and make us and keep us well Amen.

## Exercise/Prayer

- My Father my maker in heaven, I worship you. Your name be blessed and praised forever.

- ➢ I thank you for your healing power demonstrated in the bible during and after the ministry of the Lord Jesus Christ which is available for me today
- ➢ I have seen from scriptures that it is your will for me to be healed and stay in good health as it is written in **3 John 1:2** in Jesus' name.
- ➢ My Father in heaven, I believe that Jesus Christ took away sickness just as He took away sin according to **1 Peter 2:24**. His wounds bore sicknesses and diseases of all kinds, the discovered and the yet to be discovered, the curable and the incurable according to man and I therefore declare I am healed already. My body is well and no sickness or disease shall have a place in my body from this moment in Jesus' name.
- ➢ I declare so and it is so in Jesus' name. Amen

# Chapter Four

# God of all flesh - Key #4

The bible tells us through Jeremiah 32:29 that "*I am the God of all flesh, is there anything too hard for me*". You know God created everything (**John 1:3**) and that's one of the things we should meditate on seriously and see Him as the God who can never fail to repair anything because He made everything in the first place. Even car manufactures do make spare parts for the cars they manufacture and can restore damaged ones to look just as though they weren't. Now let us go back to Jeremiah 32:29 where we see God asking the question "**I am the God of all flesh, is there anything too hard for me**". God wants you to provide the answer to this question. Can anything be hard for the maker of our lives? There are several sicknesses and diseases around the world some of which man hasn't found cure for yet (medically) but we should know that with God, nothing is too hard. Here I just want to praise and exalt God. I cannot even manage to explain His size and His power. He is magnificent, powerful and creator of all. You cannot report Him to anyone and cannot be summoned by anyone. He is God and creator of all. He created us all and has power to take away life and give life (Deut 32:39, 1 Samuel 2:26).

Can anything be too hard for the creator? Absolutely no. Luke 1:37 says "***For with God nothing shall be impossible***". This is what we are talking about, God can do anything. It is possible he can heal any disease, can keep you sickness free in Jesus' name hallelujah!

***Exercise/Prayer***

- ➢ My Father my maker in heaven, I worship you. Your name be blessed and praised forever.
- ➢ You're the God that made everyone and you cannot fail to heal any disease

- I therefore pray that every cell in my body respond to your word in my mouth as I declare my body healed in Jesus' name.
- My Father in heaven the God of all flesh, I declare in the name of Jesus Christ that cells in my body be repaired to functions the way you created them, abnormal growths disappear, diseased body organs be recreated, missing body parts appear in the name of Jesus Christ by whom all things were made I pray.
- I declare so and it is so in Jesus' name. Amen

## Chapter Five

## Faith - Key #5

The subject of faith in the bible is one of the most important we can ever learn about for without it, we cannot please God and actually everything of God in the spirit realm are accessed by faith.  Faith as defined by the bible is actually ***the substance of things hoped for and an evidence of things not seen*** (Hebrews 11:1). This is very important for us to grasp in our spirit. I will straight away begin to refer to healing. When someone is sick, there might be pain, growths and any other symptoms and in the natural, that is what a person feels and see. Now when healing is desired from God, faith is necessary because by it, spiritual activations take place, causing manifestations to happen in this natural world. When a person is sick, what is hoped for is healing, recovery from pain and any disease. Therefore what is needed in the first place is the possession of necessary faith which is a substance and evidence of the unseen healing. The healing will follow faith, they go together just like any other miracles anyone might need, they all go together with faith. Therefore if you have necessary faith for healing, you have the healing.

Now you may be asking how you can have this necessary faith, well we know the bible in Romans 10:17 says "***faith comes by hearing and hearing by the word of God***'. You must make sure you read scriptures where the bible describes people being healed as well as where God has promised healing. As you read these scriptures meditatively, you will receive faith which with make you bold and assured of the healing.

God's word when received gives birth to faith in your spirit and all of the sudden, you begin to have an assurance that the sickness is gone, you begin to see yourself out of the sick bed, the pain is gone you begin to have a feeling of boldness within you that prompts you to begin to speak spontaneous words of authority over your health. You may also get prompted to take some acts of faith such as rising up if you were laying down, getting up from a wheelchair etc depending on the condition. When this happens to you, sometimes healing angles or the Lord Jesus himself could be around you in the spirit realm ministering to you as you're declaring and doing such acts.

Mark 11:24 says "***Therefore I tell you, whatever you ask for in prayer, believe that you have received it, and it will be yours***". Here Jesus gave a key to experiencing results when we pray which is "**believing you have received immediately you pray**". Simply believing you have received makes the difference between those who are healed and those that are not. Believing you have received makes the healing actualize. You must believe it has happened and don't be like those who are uncertain, they don't know what will happen next because their focus is on the report the doctor gave.

Our Lord Jesus through the scripture has taught us how things are done for us according to our faith. God the Father through the power of the Holy Spirit and His angels perform God's commands according to our faith. Let me give a few more examples we should learn this from. Mathews 8:13 **_"Then Jesus said to the centurion, "Go! As you have believed, so will it be done for you_. _And his servant was healed at that very hour_"** For me this is straight forward and we should not find it difficult to experience God's power for our health. As you have believed, so shall God do things for you! The question you should be asking yourself now is "**what have I believed?**" For those that don't believe in miracles so shall it be for them they will see none. But for people like me who believe in miracles, we experience them. These men and women recorded in the bible had some of the most difficult issues, however through their faith in Jesus, power was released to heal them. The same will happen today for anyone. See also Mathew 9:29 which says "**_Then he touched their eyes,_** *saying, "According to your faith be it done to you"* According to your faith, cancer, HIV, or any other disease can die in Jesus' name. My prayer is that this book increases and activates necessary faith in you for your miracle or to be used by God to help others. I have so much boldness when I pray to God because of my belief, my faith in Him. He cannot lie, only speaks the truth and again Jesus said "I am the way, the truth and life" and therefore all He said in His word is truth

Another wonderful scripture about faith is Mark 5:34 which says "*He said to her, "Daughter, your faith has healed you. Go in peace and be freed from your suffering"* This woman in this passage of scripture was not prayed for by the Lord Jesus for her to be healed. She drew the healing power of God from Jesus' body by touching the hem of His garment. Read this story from verse 25 so that you can see how it all happened. What made the healing power of God to flow was her faith. Verse 25 says "*because she thought, "If I just touch his clothes, I will be healed."* And in verse 29 she was immediately healed of the flow of blood she suffered for about 12 years without anyone praying for her but only her faith. This is one of my favorite scriptures about faith for it shows how you can easily receive any miracle.

Let me also discuss James 5:15 which says "***This prayer made in faith will heal the sick; the Lord will restore them to health, and the sins they have committed will be forgiven***" Whether you're the one needing healing of maybe you're praying for the sick, the key given here is that your prayer must be a prayer of faith. What is a prayer of faith? When you go back to Mark 11:24 which we have already discussed above, you see Jesus teaching about the prayer of faith. He said "***Therefore I tell you, whatever you ask for in prayer, believe that you have received it, and it will be yours***". When you pray this kind of prayer, your thoughts will change. You won't worry anymore and you will be calm without being anxious. No matter how you feel whether you still see the symptoms or not, maintain your position after prayer and In-fact if you have faith when you pray, you will not even look for an encouragement to keep trusting in God but the faith itself within you makes you sure, bold and confident that the God of all flesh has done it.

### *Exercise/Prayer*

- ➢ My Father my maker in heaven, I worship you. Your name be blessed and praised forever.
- ➢ Lord help my faith every day to grow and to be exercised according to your will/word.
- ➢ Lord this is my faith right now that I am healed, I will not be sick, I rise up right now from the bed of affliction in the name of Jesus Christ.
- ➢ Healing and good health is my potion and not sickness and disease. This is my position
- ➢ In Jesus' name I pray and it is so Amen.

# Chapter Six

# Authority - Key #6

Now authority is the legal right and power to give orders that control others' opinions, decisions, judgments and behavior. And what I am saying here that through the use of spiritual authority, you can give orders against sickness.  Reading from Luke 10:19 the bible says "***I have given you authority to trample on snakes and scorpions and to overcome all the power of the enemy; nothing will harm you***". This is the legal right we are talking about here to give orders that control the works and plans of the devil. It is the devil who afflicts people with sicknesses and diseases and we as believers have been given authority over him. In Acts 10:38, we read about **God anointing Jesus Christ of Nazareth with the Holy Spirit and power to heal all that were oppressed of the devil**. Therefore we must command and order sickness which is one of the manifestations of the works of the devil to be flashed out of the body in Jesus' name. You must also know that satanic works are forceful and therefore we exercise authority with a command and not like you're making a request.  It's non-negotiable and we have to exercise our legal right by casting out the devils behind the suffering in command form until satan let go. **Mark 16:17-18** Jesus said we can cast out devils in His name and heal the sick. As a believer in Christ Jesus, you have the legal right to exercise authority over demons and sickness using the name of Jesus Christ and therefore you need to have confidence as you give commands.

Let u look at a few examples in the scriptures about authority in action. Mathew 8:5 – 10, 13 "***When Jesus had entered Capernaum, a centurion came and pleaded with Him, "Lord, my servant lies at home, paralyzed and in terrible agony." "I will go and heal him," Jesus replied. The centurion answered, "Lord, I am not worthy to have You come*** *under my roof. But just say the word, and my servant will be healed. For I myself am a man under authority, with soldiers under me. I tell one to go, and he goes; and another to come, and he comes. I tell my servant to do something, and he does it." When Jesus heard this, He marveled and said to those following Him, "Truly I tell you, I have not found anyone in Israel with such great faith."*

This man was a soldier and he understood how authority works. He was a man who gave orders to his servants and they obeyed whatever he said and therefore thought to himself Jesus has authority as well over anything and He can just command the sickness to go and it shall go without coming over to my house!. This is another amazing story about faith and authority in the bible. Verse 13 says

*"Then Jesus said to the centurion, "Go! Let it be done just as you believed it would." And his servant was healed at that moment"*

Through this scripture, we learn how we can use and exercise orders against sickness. You have the authority as a Christian that awaits you to exercise it and the devil knows that and that's why he works hard to give Christians doubt and fear to cripple them In terms of exercising authority. In order for you to use your authority over the enemy, you need to be bold and firm knowing that you are using authentic and legal right to demand obedience to what you're saying or commanding. Jesus said ***"Then Jesus came to them and said, "All authority in heaven and on earth has been given to Me. Therefore go and make disciples of all nations, baptizing them in the name of the Father, and of the Son, and of the Holy Spirit***" (Mathew 28:18-19). Such authority our Lord Jesus exercised over devils, sicknesses and diseases was delegated to us the believers in Him. We operate in His name and therefore we should know it's not about our power but His. And that's why satan is no much for us, no sickness can resist our words because we don't speak from ourselves but legally exercise the authority of God delegated to us Hallelujah!

James 4:7 says "***Submit yourselves, then, to God. Resist the devil, and he will flee from you***" So many people are crying and feeling pity on themselves because of how they have suffered at the hands of the devil instead of rising up to resist that sickness, disease and suffering. God's word is truth and that's where we get our confidence. It is written "**the devil will flee**" because of our resistance to him and his powers. Lastly but not the least on using authority against sickness, let me add the story of Peter's mother in-law. Luke 4:38 – 39 "***After Jesus had left the synagogue, He went to the home of Simon, whose mother-in-law was suffering from a high fever. So they appealed to Jesus on her behalf, So he bent over her and rebuked the fever, and it left her. She got up at once and began to wait on them***" I looked at 25 different bible versions on this and I discovered about 20 versions used the word "**rebuked**", 3 versions used the word "**ordered**" and 2 used the word "**commanded**". All these three words show us the use of authority over the fever Peter's mother in-law had. As we use the name of Jesus against sickness, we are to rebuke, order and command sickness just as Jesus did it. The fever left her because Jesus rebuked, ordered and commanded it to leave. You can command cancer, HIV or any sickness to leave the body in the name of Jesus Christ and it shall be so in Jesus' name. Remember that when we are commanding sickness, we stand in the shoes of Jesus Christ as we use His name which has power to make satan bow. Philippians 2:9-10 says "***Therefore God exalted Him to the highest place and gave Him the name above all names, that at the name of Jesus every knee should bow, in heaven and on earth and under the earth***". As we use the name of Jesus, we must have this in our imagination that every kneel bows at the name of Jesus. One of the reasons I have so much boldness and faith when I exercise authority over satan is because I know that it's not my own authority but that of Jesus Christ. So When I command, order and rebuke the enemy, I don't have to worry whether it will work or not because it's not my ability I use but it's actually Jesus doing it through me and that's the main reason sickness, disease and demonic bondages die.


## *Exercise/Prayer*

- ➢ My Father my maker in heaven, I worship you. Your name be blessed and praised forever.
- ➢ Lord I thank you for the authority you have given me in the name of Jesus Christ.
- ➢ Right now my father God in heaven I take authority over every sickness and disease in my body and I command by body to healed now in Jesus' name.
- ➢ I command every spirit behind the pain, the sickness and disease to leave the body right now in the name of Jesus Christ
- ➢ Sickness and disease leave right now in the name of Jesus Christ.

➢ I declare so and It is so in Jesus' name

# Chapter Seven

# Love and Forgiveness - Key #7

It is very important for us to understand how love and forgiveness are connected to our health. 1Corinthians 13:13 says "***And now these three remain: faith, hope and love. But the greatest of these is love***". We must all possess love for God and for other people in this world and I have seen it as a catalyst when it comes to prayer. God is all about love and we have no reason to fail to love as well if we are Christians. According to this scripture, love is greater than everything else including hope and faith and that's one thing God will always look for in any person's actions. Do you have a love motivation behind your prayers and actions? Forgiveness is when you let go of the feelings of resentment against someone that hurt you and its cardinal you gladly do that. During our crossover night of prayer from 31st Dec 2019 to 1st Jan 2020, I felt the Lord lead me to give 12 things people need to remember they do in this new year which included "**love every day**" and "**forgive everyday**". These 2 things cannot just happen automatically but you have to deliberately decide to love and forgive even before you're hurt by anyone. Everyday make it to be in your thoughts, even as you go to bed, ask yourself "**am I feeling hurt and angry or bitter against anyone**?" The bible says "***Be angry and do not sin; do not let the sun go down on your anger***" so for sure a person might hurt you and u might also be angry but God says don't sin. When you're hurt and you fail to forgive, you sin and this will short circuit the flow of God's healing power. Let me tell prophetically that so many people are not healed today because of the anger, bitterness in their hearts. They have unsettled issues of hurt with other people and have vowed to pay evil for evil. You cannot be healed like that. Show me a man who lives in good health and I will show you a man of love, a man who easily let go of the anger. I have ministered prayer to so many people and I have seen many bitter hearts and yet they desire God to have mercy, compassion on them and heal them

In Mark 11:24 – 25 Jesus said "**24 Therefore I tell you, whatever you ask for in prayer, believe that you have received it, and it will be yours. 25 And when you stand praying, if you hold anything against anyone, forgive them, so that your Father in heaven may forgive you your sins**." Here we see Jesus connecting answers to prayer with forgiveness. This is very clear here, if you don't forgive, you won't be forgiven of your wrongs which you commit every day. There are so many wrong things we commit everyday such that sometimes we are not even conscious of. If you're not forgiven by God, you can't access healing. I heard a story of a woman who was healed of a goiter just after she let go of the hurt she had against another woman. The goiter disappeared immediately she hugged the woman she was angry with.

Let me add one last scripture on this; Mathew 5:23-25 "***Therefore if you are offering your gift at the altar and there remember that your brother has something against you, leave your gift there in front of the altar. First go and be reconciled to them; then come and offer your gift Reconcile quickly with your adversary, while you are still on the way to court. Otherwise he may hand you over to the judge, and the judge may hand you over to the officer, and you may be thrown into prison***" God demands we approach His thrown with hearts that are free of bitterness. He says you must leave the gift on the altar and be reconciled first with your brother/sister. Meaning if you don't do that, your gift may not be accepted before God. That gift Jesus was talking about also stands for worship you want to offer, a prayer, a petition or prayer request you may be wanting to offer before God's altar. This is how important love and forgiveness are. God wants us to live at peace with everyone and in fact in **Hebrews 12:14** it is written ***"Make every effort to live in peace with everyone and to be holy; without holiness no one will see the Lord'***. It's not every person you can live at peace with, however what God will mark is your effort. Therefore leaving the gift on the altar to seek reconciliation first with another person is effort. If the other person doesn't want to have anything to do with you, at least you sincerely made effort. So please go ahead let go of every anger. I have to be blunt as I encourage you here for you cannot access God's healing power when you hate some people. Please let go, forgive and talk to God about it if it seems heavy for you. The Holy Spirit will help you. There is no time I asked for the help of Holy Spirit when I wasn't helped.

### Exercise/Prayer

> My Father my maker in heaven, I worship you. Your name be blessed and praised forever.

- ➢ Lord I take this moment to forgive every person that hurt me. I forgive because I know I need your forgiveness as well in Jesus 'name

- ➢ Lord help me to love every person I have had been bitter against. When I see them I choose to feel your love about them therefore Lord give me your grace to live life like this every day in Jesus' name I pray Amen.

# Chapter Eight

## Atmosphere - Key #8

Another way to access healing is by being in an atmosphere of God's manifest presence. There are different presences of God but here I am talking about the manifest presence of God's power evidenced by miracles that take place. An atmosphere of God's presence can be created by a number of things we can do and also by being in the presence of people that carry an active presence of God's power. There are people who carry the presence of God's power that is active 24/7 and when you're in their presence, you can receive any miracle by the power of the Holy Spirit.

### Atmosphere around anointed men

Let me encourage you with a few biblical examples of men who carried atmospheres of God's manifest presence. First lets us look at the son of man the Lord Jesus Himself as an example because though

He was still God on earth, he was also human. Luke 5:17 "***And it came to pass on a certain day, as he was teaching, that there were Pharisees and doctors of the law sitting by, which were come out of every town of Galilee, and Judaea, and Jerusalem: and the power of the Lord was present to heal them***". In this meeting the Lord Jesus held, there was an atmosphere of God's healing power. It was a charged up atmosphere and people where just getting healed and testifying of the goodness of God. He carried the atmosphere that blessed people with healings and deliverances. The same atmosphere made certain people repent of their sins and became believers. Many sort to touch him, see him to just look at him, such an awe.  In **Acts 5:15-16** we read "***15 As a result, people brought the sick into the streets and laid them on beds and mats so that at least Peter's shadow might fall on some of them as he passed by. 16 Crowds gathered also from the towns around Jerusalem, bringing their sick and*** *those tormented by impure spirits, and all of them were healed"*. Peter had such an atmosphere of God's power around him such that people even thought it was his shadow that was healing them because they noticed that whenever they came within the proximity of his shadow, miracles were happening to them. It was an atmosphere that was charged up with God's power that healed and delivered people from demonic torments. **Acts 11:15** says "*As I began to speak,*" Peter continued, "*the Holy Spirit fell on them, just as he fell on us at the beginning*" Peter carried a great anointing at this time because as you can see him testifying here, the Spirit of God manifested and came upon everyone without Peter praying for them. He said he just started speaking and not praying. I have people testify in my ministry of how they got healed by just entering church. On a certain Sunday, one young lady was giving a testimony of how she got healed when I just greeted her. That's all about the goodness and faithfulness of God.

## Atmosphere during prayer and worship

The healing power of God can come upon people during worship. When you worship God, you create an atmosphere that even angels love to be in. The angels that are earth are attracted to such moments and people present can begin to experience God's power. In **Acts 13:1** we read "**1** *Now in the church at Antioch there were prophets and teachers: Barnabas, Simeon called Niger, Lucius of Cyrene, Manaen (who had been brought up with Heroɑ the tetrarch) and Saul. 2 While they were worshiping the Lord and fasting, the Holy Spirit said, "Set apart for me Barnabas and Saul for the work to which I have called them*" They prayed, fasted, and ministered to God through worship and this created an atmosphere for God to minister to them. Here we read about God ministering to them in form of an instruction however it can also be in form of God healing and performing miracles among people because the atmosphere is ready for the supernatural to step in.

Let me also talk about the story of Paul and Silas found in **Acts 16**. I will just talk about verses 25 and 26 but you can still read the whole chapter just to enjoy the full story. My interest on this discussion starts from verse 25 through to 26 which says "**25 *And at midnight Paul and Silas prayed, and sang praises unto God: and the prisoners heard them. And suddenly there was a great earthquake, so that the foundations of the prison were shaken: and immediately all the doors were opened, and every one's bands were loosed*'** These two men through prayer and the songs they sang created an atmosphere that broke the chains used to bind them. As you pray for your health, worship God, sing songs of praise and worship that will help create the atmosphere for God to work and please choose songs wisely i.e right songs that will invite such a mighty power of God for healing and deliverance. I say choose songs wisely because not every nice song is a right song. Some songs sound nice but aren't consistent with God's word and therefore, will not attract angelic visitation and God's power.

So I encourage you to create an atmosphere of God's manifest presence through praying, fasting and worshiping God. You can't carry God's healing power when you're always with cold and lukewarm people, always listening to worldly music. There is music you can listen to that just charges up the atmosphere around you with God's power and healing angels.

### *Exercise*

> Be in Church or in the presence of anointed men and women of God

> Be in an atmosphere of praise and worship or you can create that atmosphere yourself by beginning to worship God every day and listening to great worship music

## Chapter Nine

## God's word - Key #9

Did you know that whatever God does, He does it by sending His word first? How was this whole world created? Hebrews 11:3 says "**By faith we understand that the universe was created by the word of God, so that what is seen was not made out of things that are visible**" therefore you must know that there is creative power in God's word. You must always learn to release God's word over your health i.e confessing what God's word has said as you shall see in the examples I have given in the prayer below. **Jeremiah 1:12** says "**Then the LORD said to me, "You have seen well, for I am watching over my word to perform it**" God has promised to do what His word says and if you keep speaking what He has said over your health, you will see His power in action.

In Psalms 103:20 we read "***Bless the LORD, O you his angels, you mighty ones who do his word, obeying the voice of his word***". Angels obey God's word and if you're going to be releasing God's word over your situation, you will be releasing angels of God also and that's how you can receive angelic help by the way in any situation. In Psalms 107:20 it is written "***He sent out his word and healed them; he rescued them from the grave***" There is healing power in God's word and what you need is to meditate on it by **reading it over and over, thinking about it over and over** and **speaking it into your life or situation over and over**. That's what meditations is all about. Some people think meditation is only being quiet and thinking. The Latin word from which meditation comes has several meaning to it which includes, *reflecting, acting, studying* and *talking*. God's word in Hebrews 4:12 says "***For the word of God is alive and active. Sharper than any double-edged sword, it penetrates even to dividing soul and spirit, joints and marrow; it*** *judges the thoughts and attitudes of the heart"* With the word of God you can cut off any sickness from your body. It's a sword that is shaper than anything. God's word can go where doctors may not go for it will remove even the spiritual causes of diseases. I have seen sick people who when they went to the hospital, the doctors found nothing wrong with them. I have seen God heal people that tried all medical efforts to treat and yet no improvements were realized.

## Exercise/Prayer

- My Father my maker in heaven, I worship you. Your name be blessed and praised forever.
- Lord I believe by faith that through your word, the worlds were created and I speak such power to create over my body right now to recreate dead cells and diseased body organs in Jesus' name
- I speak the creative power of God over my body right now in the name of Jesus Christ.

- ➢ Father in heaven like you said "let there light and there was light", I also declare let there be healing in my body right now in Jesus' name
- ➢ I declare so and it is so in the Jesus' name Amen.

## Chapter Ten

## Your Mouth - Key #10

Did you know that most of the problems many people have today are because of their own words? There are people who never committed a crime but are imprisoned on account of their own words while some criminals are out there free because of how they talked in the courts of law either through a lawyer or by themselves.

Let us start by looking as **Proverbs 18:20-21** which says "***From the fruit of his mouth a man's belly is filled; with the harvest from his lips he is satisfied. Life and death are in the power of the tongue, and those who love it will eat its fruit***" You know what? I don't like to complicate things of God when they are not complicated in the first place. It is written here where life and death are activated and it's in the power of the tongue! Do you want sickness to die? Use your tongue! Do you want your body to live and not die of sickness? Use your tongue and that's how God has made it easy for us hallelujah! We all eat the fruits of our mouths i.e what we say! **Romans 10:10** says "***For with the heart man believeth unto righteousness; and with the mouth confession is made unto salvation***" What the mouth confesses must be what the heart has believed. So many people are still sick because there is no Godly faith in them so they only confess doubt and are not certain whether they will be healed or not. If you believe, use your mouth to confess your healing and good health. If you are not sick, still you need to confess your good health out. By the grace of God I am a beneficiary of God's grace such that I don't get sick and you know what? I confess my good health out loud with my mouth from time to time and it works for me. Don't wait until sickness knocks to start praying and confessing you're well.

2 Corinthians 4:13 puts it this way; "***It is written:
"I believed; therefore I have spoken." Since
we have that same spirit of faith, we also
believe and therefore speak***" You can only be
speaking out loud what you believe are confident
about. For instance, some Christians aren't even
bold enough to declare they are going to heaven.
Don't fear to declare out loud what you have
believed concerning anything which of course
includes healing which is the main subject in this
book. I will be so glad to hear your testimony of
how you have been healed, staying in good health
or even how God will be using you to heal the sick.

Look also at Mark 11:13-14 which says "***Seeing in
the distance a fig tree in leaf, He went to see
if there was any fruit on it. But when He
reached it, He found nothing on it except
leaves, since it was not the season for figs,
May no one ever eat fruit from you again."
And his disciples heard him say it***" Jesus here
talks to a tree as though he was speaking to a
human being. People are accustomed to thinking

they can only speak to humans or God or even anything that would respond to them in form of words or sound, however here Jesus demonstrated another powerful key to effect changes in our lives as believers in Christ. The story didn't end there because the following day something everyone could see has happened to the tree Jesus spoke to. When He spoke to it no one saw any change except His disciples hearing him speak to the tree and wondering what was happening. Verses 20 – 23 says "***In the morning, as they went along, they saw the fig tree withered from the roots. 21 Peter remembered and said to Jesus, "Rabbi, look! The fig tree you cursed has withered!"22 "Have faith in God," Jesus answered. 23 "Truly[a] I tell you, if anyone says to this mountain, 'Go, throw yourself into the sea,' and does not doubt in their heart but believes that what they say will happen, it will be done for them***" Wow! The tree had dried up and the disciples were shocked! And the Lord just responded **"have faith in God"** and then He added the principle of using the month to move anything.  By faith, you can use your mouth to speak to the sickness to move out of body and Jesus said it will happen. I would rather believe Jesus and I do so. He is creator the bible says all things where made by him and I am safe when I believe in Jesus Christ my savior.

### *Exercise/Prayer*

> My Father my maker in heaven, I worship you. Your name be blessed and praised forever.

> Just as the Lord Jesus cursed the fig tree and it dried up, I engage the same power right now to work for me.

> In the name of Jesus Christ I command any sickness and disease in my body to die right now.

> From today I declare that I will never be sick again in Jesus' name

> I declare so and it is so in Jesus' name

## Chapter Eleven

## My Testimony

I just want to share with you one or two testimonies about how the Lord has been faithful to His word in my life. If you use these simple keys I have shared with you in this book, you too will see God's healing power in your life and even through your life to others. I remember when I was younger I used to get sick so much but thank God He preserved my life even when I didn't know Him the way I do now. The first example I will give is back in 1995 when I had severe eye problem. Let me first give you a brief background about this. Around 1988 or 1989 a snake spit into my eyes and I don't really know if the eye problem I developed after about 6 years or so was caused by this incidence. However, in 1995, I had a doctor recommend the type of lens for me to wear because of my sight which had become bad. My eyes kept itching every day and would often get swollen. When I was In secondary school, I sometimes couldn't see what the teach wrote on the black board, except seeing some kind of whitish or milky stuff until after a few seconds or so when I would see notes again on the board. This was affecting me so much even in my academics. My dad couldn't buy the glasses the doctor recommended for reasons I didn't know, however, I was daily applying medicines such as eyes drops and so on. But a time came when my faith in the Lord God began to increase rapidly and I just began to believe God for good health. I began to see myself with good sight and not blind, in good health and not sick. This was going on within my imagination by faith because of the impact of God's word and the Holy Spirit on my mind and spirit. Today I have very perfect sight all by God's grace and power through faith and I don't wear lenses for eye problems. That problem disappeared just like that i.e by faith in Christ Jesus.

One day in 2007, I remember feeling feverish and I was really feeling very bad. I rushed to read a scripture which I have shared already in one of the chapters and I want you to hold on to that scripture all your life. I use this scripture to declare continuous good health till Jesus our Lord comes. 1 Peter 2:24 says "***He Himself bore our sins in His body on the tree, so that we might die to sin and live to righteousness. By His stripes you are healed***" This is in past tense and it just makes me bold about declaring myself in good health for I have already been healed through the wounds of my Lord Jesus. Therefore sickness has no place in my body. If you're a believer in Christ Jesus, believe this and take your good health right now. Jesus took the sickness, the diseases just as He took the sins. Cancer, HIV, malaria, diabetics and any other sickness and disease have no place in your body unless the place you give them through ignorance, sin, unbelief and negative confessions.

Another day came when I had some sores on my back which were so painful. I was so much in pain such that bending over was a very big problem. I went to the hospital where I was given a plastic bag full of medicines. When I got home, I took the medicine so that I can drink and apply some on the sores and then just before I did that, I remembered that I had been praying to God that I will not take any medicine that year. I began to pray about my health when I was well in my body and so now my faith was being tested when these sores came on my body. Can you guess what I did after remembering my prayer? I immediately put away the medicine by faith and I straight away spoke healing over my body by faith. I said within myself that taking the medication was going to cancel the prayer I had been praying all that year. I believed God had answered my prayer and that He was going to keep me from anything that would harm my body to cause me to take medication. I prayed

prayers of prevention and that was it. I have
never been sick since that year and I have
never taken medicine since that year. It's been
years now. Am I special as in being better than
other people? Absolutely not. What works for
me can work for anyone and that's why I am
sharing this information in this little book so
that people can live in good health. I hate
sickness and by faith I believe God has given
me grace to pray against it. I have seen God
heal people of different sicknesses and
diseased and you too God can keep strong and
in good health.

**Clarification/Caution**; Taking medication is
good, when I say I stopped taking medication, it's
because I have built my faith over time. It didn't
happen overnight but I constantly eat the scriptures
such that an unusual boldness and faith was
birthed in me that makes me resist sickness. So if
you're taking medicine, please continue for it is by
faith through the real work of the Holy Spirit that

God can take you to another level. However God can also speak to you on what to do. I still encourage people to go to the hospital and take medicine doctors prescribe until they are instructed to stop. When we pray for people, we also encourage them to get tested at the hospital. I have heard of people who died because they stopped taking ARVs for HIV by themselves or because immature ministers told them not to continue drinking because they prayed. So I have to clarify and caution you here.

So be encouraged that Jesus was never sick and we have access to the same blessing of good health. I can also give you testimonies of people God has healed after I prayed with them however, I thought I just share with you how I have responded to sickness so that you too can be encouraged and begin to build your faith which will not only benefit you but also the people around you. I have also had people in my ministry come to testify how sickness began to be scarce in their lives and families by simply submitting to me in ministry. I humbly thank God almighty for this grace.

**Let me pray for you**; I pray to my heavenly Father my maker the God of all flesh. I pray that God bless you, heal you, keep you in good health and use you to heal others in the name of Jesus Christ. I decree an impartation of compassion and healing anointing in your life in Jesus' name I decree over your life Amen.

## About the Author

Apostle Arthur Musonda is an author, speaker, gospel singer, song writer, music teacher and Founder of **The Residence of Christ Ministries**. He is a Minster of the word with a passion for sharing God's word on subjects that will change the practical daily lives of listeners and readers. He also holds a Bachelor of Divinity degree, an Associate of Divinity Degree, Diploma of Ministry, Diploma of Divinity and a Commissioned Pastoral Diploma and runs a Prophetic, Healing and Deliverance Ministry which is dedicated to make known to humanity what God is saying in these last days.

**The Residence of Christ Ministries** headquarters is in Mkushi Zambia running two services on Sundays. The morning services are from 08:00hrs to 12:30hrs (8am to 12:30pm) and the Prophetic, Deliverance and Healing Service in the afternoons runs from 13:00hrs to 16:00hrs (1pm to 4pm). All these services and mainly run by Apostle Arthur Musonda.

Contact us **on +260 977 497010**,

*arthur4heaven@yahoo.com*

Connection on Facebook

***https://web.facebook.com/profile.php?id=545***
***998052596043&ref=br_rs***

If you would like to ask the Apostle to come and speak in your meetings or conferences please you can contact him or the co-ordinator using the above details.